TITLE
CANCER REMISSION

SUBTITLE
How to cure cancer fast, nutrition and diet for a cancer free life

Author name
Dr James Brandon

INTRODUCTION

In most people's perceptions, there is no worse diagnosis than that of cancer. Cancer is frequently conceived as being an untreatable, terribly painful illness with no cure. However widespread this perspective of cancer may be, it is overblown and overgeneralized.

Cancer is a severe and even life-threatening condition. For example, it is the top cause of death among Americans under the age of 80 and the second highest cause of death among older Americans. There will be 1.5 million new cases of cancer in the United States next year, with over 570,000 deaths as a result of not including basal and squamous cell skin cancers, which are not recorded but could add another two million cases each year (ACS, 2010). (ACS, 2010).

However, it is a mistake to suppose that all kinds of cancer are untreatable and lethal.

The fact of the problem is that there are various varieties of cancer, many of which can now be properly treated to eradicate, diminish, or delay the effects of the illness on patients' lives. While a cancer diagnosis may still leave people feeling powerless and out of control, in many situations nowadays there is a reason for optimism rather than despair.

Our purpose in this area is to educate you on the fundamentals of cancer and cancer therapy. Possessing this information will, we hope, assist you to understand better what cancer is, how it arises, and how to make educated decisions regarding cancer treatment alternatives.

Chapter 1: CANCER?

Your body is composed of many millions of tiny cells, each a self-contained living unit. Normally, each cell coordinates with the others that compose tissues and organs of your body. One way that this coordination occurs is reflected in how your cells reproduce themselves. Normal cells in the body grow and divide for a period of time and then stop growing and dividing. Thereafter, they only reproduce themselves as necessary to replace defective or dying cells. Cancer occurs when this cellular reproduction process goes out of control. In other words, cancer is a disease characterized by uncontrolled, uncoordinated and undesirable cell division. Unlike normal cells, cancer cells continue to grow and divide for their whole lives, replicating into more and more harmful cells.

The abnormal growth and division observed in cancer cells is caused by damage in these cells' DNA (genetic material inside cells that determines cellular characteristics and functioning). There are a variety of ways that cellular DNA can become damaged and defective. For example, environmental factors (such as exposure to tobacco smoke) can initiate a chain of events that results in cellular DNA defects that lead to cancer. Alternatively, defective DNA can be inherited from your parents.

As cancer cells divide and replicate themselves, they often form into a clump of cancer cells known as a ***tumor. Tumors*** cause many of the symptoms of cancer by pressuring, crushing and destroying surrounding non-cancerous cells and tissues.

Tumors come in two forms; benign and malignant.

Benign tumors are not cancerous, thus they do not grow and spread to the extent of cancerous tumors. Benign tumors are usually not life threatening. **Malignant tumors**, on the other hand, grow and spread to other areas of the body. The process whereby cancer cells travel from the initial tumor site to other parts of the body is known as metastasis.

Chapter 2:WHAT BRINGS ON CANCER?

Mutations, or alterations to the DNA in your cells, are the primary cause of cancer. Mutations in the DNA can be inherited. In addition, they may develop later in life as a result of environmental factors.

These outside factors, often known as **carcinogens**, may consist of:

.ultraviolet light and radiation are physical carcinogens (UV) cigarette smoke, asbestos, alcohol, air pollution, tainted food, and drinking water are examples of mild chemical carcinogens.

.biological cancer-causing agents such as bacteria, viruses, and parasites

According to the WHOTrusted Source, roughly 33% of cancer-related fatalities may be related to cigarette use, alcohol usage, having a high body mass index (BMI), eating few fruits and vegetables, and not exercising enough.

RISK ELEMENTS

Your chances of getting cancer may increase if you have certain risk factors. These risk elements may consist of:

According to medical research, unhealthy diets include starchy foods, refined carbohydrates like sugars and processed grains, high alcohol and tobacco usage, red and processed meat, sugary drinks, and salty snacks.
an absence of exercise
exposure to radiation without protection
exposure to ultraviolet (UV) light from the sun infection by some viruses, such as the Epstein-Barr virus, which causes infectious

mononucleosis, H. pylori, human papillomavirus (HPV), hepatitis B, hepatitis C, HIV, and hepatitis B and C

Additionally, as people age, their risk of having cancer rises. According to the National Cancer Institute, the risk of having cancer generally rises until the age of 70 to 80 and then declines (NCI).

This could be the outcome of, according to a reliable source:

aging's less efficient cell repair systems and the accumulation of risk factors from lifetime exposure to carcinogens
Your chance of developing cancer may be impacted by certain inflammatory medical disorders that you already have. A chronic inflammatory bowel illness is ulcerative colitis.

Chapter3:SEVERITY OF CANCER

Even if they spread to other parts of the body, cancers are called for the region in which they start and the type of cell they are formed. For instance, lung cancer is still used to describe cancer that starts in the lungs and spreads to the liver.

Additionally, several clinical terms are employed for certain cancer types in general:

1. cancer called a **carcinoma** begins in the skin or the tissues that border other organs.
2. **Sarcoma** is a type of cancer that affects connective tissues like blood vessels, muscles, cartilage, and bones.

3. A malignancy of the bone marrow, which produces blood cells, **_is leukemia_**.

4. Cancers of the immune system include ***lymphoma and myeloma***.

Learn more about various kinds of cancer using the resources below.

appendix cancer
bladder cancer
bone cancer
brain cancer
breast cancer
cervical cancer
colon or colorectal cancer
duodenal cancer
ear cancer
endometrial cancer
esophageal cancer
heart cancer
gallbladder cancer
kidney or renal cancer
laryngeal cancer
leukemia
lip cancer
liver cancer

lung cancer
lymphoma
mesothelioma
myeloma\soral cancers
ovarian cancer
pancreatic cancer
penile cancer
prostate cancer
rectal cancer
skin cancer
small intestine cancer
spleen cancer
stomach or gastric cancer
testicular cancer
thyroid cancer
uterine cancer
vaginal cancer
vulvar cancer

Signs and symptoms of cancer may include:

.lumps or growths on the body.

sudden weight loss.

fever,tiredness and fatigue.

pain.

nocturnal sweats.

changes in digestion.

modifications in skin.

cough

Specific kinds of cancers often have their warning indicators.
If .you are having .unexplainable symptoms, it is .best to consult a doctor for a diagnosis.

HOW DOES CANCER GROW AND SPREAD?

Abnormal cell division

Normal cells in your body grow and divide. Each one has a life cycle determined by the sort of cell. As cells are harmed or die off, new cells take their place.

Cancer interrupts this system and leads cells to grow improperly. It's produced by abnormalities or mutations in the cell's DNA.

The DNA in each cell provides instructions that tell the cell what to do and how to grow and divide. Mutations occur commonly in DNA, but ordinarily, cells correct these abnormalities. When a mistake is not fixed, a cell could become **malignant**.

Mutations may cause cells that should be replaced to survive instead of die, and new cells to emerge when they're not necessary. These extra cells may divide unchecked, causing tumors to form.

.Creation of tumors

Tumors may produce health risks, depending on where they originate in the body.

Not all tumors are cancerous. ***Benign tumors*** are noncancerous and do not spread to nearby tissues.

But sometimes, tumors may grow enormous and produce complications when they press against neighboring organs and tissue. Cancerous tumors are ***malignant*** and may invade other sections of the body.

.Metastasis

Some cancer cells may also migrate through the circulation or lymphatic system to distant areas of the body. This is called metastasis.

Cancers that have metastasized are judged more advanced than those that have not.

Metastatic cancers are typically harder to treat and more fatal.

Chapter 4:THE IMPORTANCE OF EARLY DETECTION OF CANCER

Early detection happens when cancer is diagnosed in its early stages. This may increase the effectiveness of treatment and minimize the mortality rate.

Cancer screenings may help find indicators of cancer early. Some common cancer screenings may detect:

.Cervical cancer and prostate cancer. Some screenings, such as for cervical cancer and prostate cancer, may be done as part of routine examinations.

.Lung cancer. Screenings for lung cancer may be undertaken frequently for those who have certain risk factors.

.*Skin cancer*. Skin cancer screenings may be undertaken by a dermatologist if you have skin concerns or are at risk of skin cancer.

.*Colorectal cancer*. The American Cancer Society (ACS)Trusted Source suggests regular screenings for colorectal cancer begin at age 45. These examinations are routinely done during a colonoscopy. At-home testing kits may also be able to diagnose some forms of colorectal cancer,

.*Breast cancer*. Mammograms to screen for breast cancer are indicated for women aged 45 and older Trusted Source, although you may elect to begin tests at age 40. In those with a high risk, testing may be indicated early.

If you have a family history of cancer or have a high risk of having cancer, it is vital to follow a doctor's screening recommendations.

While recognizing cancer warning signs may help individuals with cancer seek diagnosis and treatment, many cancers may be difficult to identify early and may not exhibit symptoms until the later stages.

Chapter 5:CANCER TREATMENT

Cancer therapy may involve many alternatives, depending on the kind of cancer and how advanced it is.

.Localized therapy. Localized treatment typically entails applying therapies like surgery or local radiation therapy to a particular location of the body or tumor.

.Systemic therapy. Systemic pharmacological therapies, such as chemotherapy, targeted therapy, and immunotherapy, may influence the whole body.

.Palliative therapy. Palliative care entails alleviating health problems connected with cancer, such as difficulties breathing and discomfort.

Different cancer therapies are typically used jointly to eliminate or kill as many malignant cells as feasible.

The most prevalent kinds of therapy for cancer are:

Surgery\sSurgery eliminates as much of cancer as feasible. Surgery is typically performed in tandem with some other treatment to make sure all of the cancer cells are gone.

Chemotherapy

Chemotherapy is a sort of aggressive cancer treatment that employs drugs that are poisonous to cells to destroy rapidly proliferating cancer cells. It may be used to diminish the size of a tumor or the number of cells in your body and lessen the probability of the disease spreading.

Radiation treatment

Radiation treatment employs intense, concentrated beams of radiation to eliminate cancer cells. Radiation treatment done inside of your body is termed brachytherapy, whereas radiation therapy done outside of your body is called external beam radiation.

Stem cell (bone marrow) transplant

This therapy heals damaged bone marrow with healthy stem cells. Stem cells are undifferentiated cells that may have several activities. These transplants let physicians use larger dosages of chemotherapy to treat the malignancy. A stem cell transplant is often used to treat leukemia.

Immunotherapy (biological treatment) (biological therapy)

Immunotherapy employs your body's immune system to fight cancer cells. These medicines help your antibodies detect the disease, so they can employ your body's natural defenses to eliminate cancer cells.

Hormone treatment

Hormone treatment eliminates or prevents hormones that drive some tumors to halt cancer cells from developing. This medication is a frequent treatment for tumors that may utilize hormones to develop and spread, such as some forms of breast cancer and prostate cancer.

Targeted medication treatment

Targeted drug treatment employs medications to interfere with particular chemicals that enable cancer cells to grow and survive. Genetic testing may indicate whether you are qualified for this form of treatment. It may depend on the kind of cancer you have and the genetic alterations and molecular properties of your tumor.

Clinical trials

Clinical trials seek innovative approaches to treat cancer. This may involve assessing the efficacy of pharmaceuticals that have previously been authorized by the Food and Drug Administration (FDA) but for different reasons. It may also entail testing new medications. Clinical trials may give another alternative for patients who may have not achieved the amount of success they desired with traditional therapies. In rare situations, therapeutic therapy may be supplied for free.

Alternative medicine

Alternative medicine may be used to augment another method of therapy. It may help minimize symptoms of cancer and adverse effects of cancer therapy, including nausea, exhaustion, and discomfort.

Alternative cancer therapy might include:

acupuncture\syoga\smassage\smeditation\
srelaxation methods
Outlook
After you obtain a cancer diagnosis, your
prognosis might depend on a variety of
circumstances. These considerations may
include:

kind of cancer\sstage of cancer at
diagnosis\slocation of cancer\sage
is\sgeneral health
Prevention
Knowing the variables that lead to cancer
may help you adopt a lifestyle that
minimizes your cancer risk.

Preventive methods to minimize your chance of acquiring cancer may include:

.avoiding cigarettes and secondhand smoke\s.

minimizing your consumption of processed meats\s.

eating a diet that emphasizes mostly plant-based foods, lean meats, and healthy fats, such as the Mediterranean diet

.avoiding alcohol or drinking in moderation

.maintaining a moderate body weight and BMI

.performing frequent moderate physical exercise for 140 to 310 minutes per week

.keeping shielded from the sun by avoiding direct sun exposure and using a wide spectrum sunscreen, hat, and sunglasses\savoiding tanning beds

.being vaccinated against viral illnesses that might lead to cancer, such as hepatitis B and HPV

Meet with a doctor regularly so they can test you for different kinds of cancer. This enhances your chances of discovering any likely cancers as early as feasible.

Meet with a doctor periodically so they can test you for several forms of cancer. This raises your chances of detecting any probable malignancies as early as possible.

Chapter 6:CAN CANCER BE CURED?

Whether a person's cancer can be cured depends on the kind and stage of the disease, the sort of therapy they can undergo, and other considerations. Some malignancies are more likely to be cured than others. But each malignancy has to be treated individually. There isn't one cure for cancer.

CURE VERSUS REMISSION

A cure indicates that cancer has gone away with therapy, no further treatment is required, and the cancer is not likely to come back. Unusually, a doctor can be positive that the cancer will never come back. In most situations, it takes time to discover whether cancer could come back. But, the longer a person remains cancer free, the higher the likelihood that cancer will not come back. More typically, when therapy looks to be beneficial, physicians will describe cancer as "in remission," rather than "cured."

Remission is a period when the cancer is responding to therapy or is under control. Some individuals assume that remission indicates cancer has been cured, but that may not be the case.

In full remission, all the signs and symptoms of cancer go gone, and cancer cells can't be discovered by any testing. In partial remission, cancer decreases but doesn't go away. Remissions may last anywhere from weeks to years. Treatment may or may not continue during remission, depending on the kind of cancer. Complete remissions may carry on for years and, with time, cancer may be regarded to be cured. If the cancer returns (recurrence), another remission may be achievable with extra therapy.

What do survival numbers mean?

When informed they have cancer, many patients ask their doctor what their probability of survival is. While numerous aspects go into an answer, some statistics may aid. Statistics are statistics that explain what occurs to big groups of individuals with the same condition. Statistics cannot be applied to a single individual but may offer some notion of what to anticipate.

Here are some statistics that are used for cancer:

Survival rate: the proportion of patients who are alive at a specific period following diagnosis.

Overall survival rate: the proportion of persons with a specific kind and stage of cancer who have not died from any cause during a period following diagnosis.

Cancer (or disease)-specific survival rate:

 the percentage of people with a certain type and stage of cancer who have not died from their cancer during a set period after diagnosis.

5-year relative survival rate:

the proportion of persons who will be alive 5 years following diagnosis. It does not include people who die from other ailments. Survival rates may describe any period. However, researchers commonly examine 5-year relative survival rates.

What does it mean to be cancer survivor

There is more than one definition of a cancer survivor. Some individuals use this word to refer to everyone who has ever been diagnosed with cancer. This is what the American Cancer Society implies when we speak about survival or living as a cancer survivor.

But other individuals use the word "survivor" for someone who has finished cancer treatment. And yet some may only name a person a survivor if they had survived many years following a cancer diagnosis. Remember too, that therapy lasts longer for some individuals, and not everyone completes treatment. Some individuals may survive for many years with cancer as a chronic condition.

Others who are touched, such as family and friends, could also occasionally be termed, cancer survivors.

Being a cancer survivor means different things to different people. Some people will be cancer free after treatment but may experience late and long-term side effects of treatment. Others may be cancer free after therapy but have their cancer come back and need to be treated again. Still, others will need to continue with cancer therapy to keep their cancer under control. But everybody who has been diagnosed with cancer requires care that focuses on their requirements.

Not everyone wishes to be dubbed a cancer survivor. Each individual has the right to define their experience with cancer. So, everyone who defines themselves as a cancer survivor should be considered one.

Chapter 7: LEUKEMIA?

Leukemia is a blood malignancy caused by an increase in the number of white blood cells in your body.

Those white blood cells squeeze out the red blood cells and platelets that your body needs to remain healthy. The additional white blood cells don't operate appropriately.

LEUKEMIA SYMPTOMS

Different forms of leukemia might create different issues. You may not notice any indicators in the early stages of certain kinds. When you do have symptoms, they may include:

Weakness or fatigue
Bruising or bleeding readily
Fever or chills

Infections that are severe or keep coming
back
Pain in your bones or joints
Headaches
Vomiting
Seizures
Weight loss
Night sweats
Shortness of breath
Swollen lymph nodes or organs like your
spleen

LEUKEMIA CAUSES AND RISK FACTORS

No one knows precisely what causes
leukemia. People who have it have
particular odd chromosomes, but the
chromosomes don't cause leukemia.

You can't avoid leukemia, but some factors
may induce it. You could have an increased
risk if you:

Smoke

Are exposed to a lot of radiation or certain
substances
Had radiation treatment or chemotherapy
to treat cancer
Have a family history of leukemia
Have a genetic condition like Down
syndrome

How Does Leukemia Happen?

Blood comprises three kinds of cells: white
blood cells that fight infection, red blood
cells that deliver oxygen, and platelets that
help blood clot.

Every day, your bone marrow generates
billions of new blood cells, and most of them
are red cells. When you have leukemia, your
body generates more white cells than it
needs.

These leukemia cells can't fight infection the
way regular white blood cells do. And since
there are so many of them, they start to

impair the way your organs operate. Over time, you may not have enough red blood cells to deliver oxygen, enough platelets to clot your blood, or enough normal white blood cells to fight infection.

Chapter 8:LEUKEMIA CLASSIFICATIONS

Leukemia is categorized by how rapidly it starts and becomes worse, and by which sort of blood cell is involved.

The first category, how rapidly it develops, is split into acute and chronic leukemia.

Acute leukemia arises when most of the aberrant blood cells don't mature and can't carry out regular duties. It may turn terrible very quickly.

Chronic leukemia arises when there are some immature cells, but others are normal and can operate the way they should. It goes more slowly than acute types do.

The second category, what sort of cell is involved, is separated into ***lymphocytic and myelogenous leukemia.***

Lymphocytic (or lymphoblastic) leukemia includes bone marrow cells that become lymphocytes, a form of a white blood cells.

Myelogenous (or myeloid) leukemia includes the marrow cells that generate red blood cells, platelets, and various types of white blood cells.

TYPES OF LEUKAEMIA

The four primary kinds of leukemia are:

Acute lymphocytic leukemia (ALL). This is the most frequent kind of childhood leukemia. It may spread to your lymph nodes and central nervous system.

Acute myelogenous leukemia (AML) (AML).

This is the second most frequent type of juvenile leukemia and one of the most common kinds for adults.

Chronic Lymphocytic Leukemia (Cll). ...

This is the other most frequent kind of adult leukemia. Some forms of CLL will be stable for years and won't require therapy. But with others, your body isn't able to make regular blood cells, and you'll require therapy.

Chronic myelogenous leukemia (CML) (CML).

With this kind, you may not have significant symptoms. You may not be diagnosed with it until you undergo a standard blood test. People 65 and older have an increased risk of this kind.

Chapter 9:LEUKEMIA DIAGNOSIS

Your doctor will need to look for symptoms of leukemia in your blood or bone marrow. They may undertake tests including:

Blood testing. A complete blood count (CBC) looks at the amount and maturity of various kinds of blood cells. A blood smear searches for atypical or immature cells.

Bone marrow biopsy. This test includes marrow extracted from your pelvic bone using a long needle. It can inform your doctor what sort of leukemia you have and how serious it is.

Spinal tap. This involves fluid from your spinal cord. It may inform your doctor if the disease has spread.

Imaging testing. Things like CT, MRI, and PET scans may discover symptoms of leukemia.

LEUKEMIA TREATMENTS
Can Leukemia Be Cured?

While there is presently no cure for leukemia, it is feasible to treat the illness to prevent it from coming back.

The therapy you receive depends on the kind of leukemia you have, how far it's spread, and how healthy you are. The primary possibilities are:

.Chemotherapy.

Radiation.

Biologic therapy.

Targeted therapy.

Stem cell transplant.

Surgery

.***Chemotherapy employs*** chemicals to eliminate cancer cells in your blood and bone marrow. You can obtain the medicine:

Through an injection into a vein or muscle As a pill Into the fluid surrounding your spinal cord.

Radiation employs high-energy X-rays to destroy leukemia cells or block them from developing. You may have it all over or in just one place of your body where there are a lot of cancer cells.

Biologic treatment, often termed immunotherapy, helps your immune system detect and fight cancer cells. Drugs like interleukins and interferon may help improve your body's natural defenses against leukemia.

Targeted treatment employs medications to inhibit particular genes or proteins that cancer cells require to develop. This therapy can inhibit the signals that leukemia cells use to grow and proliferate, cut off their blood supply, or kill them directly.

A stem cell transplant replaces the leukemia cells in your bone marrow with new ones that generate blood. Your doctor may receive the fresh stem cells from your own body or a donor. First, you'll get heavy doses of chemotherapy to eliminate the cancer cells in your bone marrow. Then, you'll obtain the fresh stem cells via an injection into one of your veins. They will develop into new, healthy blood cells.

.Surgery. Your doctor may remove your spleen if it's loaded with cancer cells and is pushing on adjacent organs. This treatment is termed a splenectomy.

Treatment might continue for many months or even years, depending on the kind and severity of the ailment.

SEEKING SUPPORT FOR LEUKEMIA

Receiving a leukemia diagnosis is life-altering and hard for both a person and their loved ones.

It is usual to have a combination of emotions following a cancer diagnosis, but everyone responds differently in these circumstances. Some may attempt to put on a brave façade to shield their loved ones, while others may openly seek help.

It is crucial to remember that help is accessible to everyone from a broad variety of sources, including:

Oncology care team: Asking questions about leukemia, its symptoms, treatment choices, stages, and survival statistics may help a person understand their disease.

Friends and family: Friends and family may give personal and emotional support. They may also aid a person with ordinary duties that may become too tough owing to leukemia symptoms or therapy.

Support groups: These groups are beneficial for individuals to meet others who can give advice and support from their own lived experience or expertise. Support groups exist for both those with leukemia and their loved ones.

Charities: Organizations, such as the Leukemia and Lymphoma Society, are committed to offering assistance to persons with a cancer diagnosis.

There may also be local charities and internet services that may assist a person to understand and manage their disease.

Chapter 10:HEALTHY DIETS FOR CANCER(LEUKAEMIA)

Leukemia and its therapies may have a substantial influence on the body. People who have leukemia may benefit from a diet including particular foods, enabling the body to replenish blood and tissue cells lost during cancer treatment\ssupporting the immune system\shelping the person retains or restore their strength\sreducing the chance of complications.

Types of food to consume

The LLS suggests a diet for those who have leukemia should include:

a variety of vegetables and legumes, which should make up approximately 50% of most meals\sentire fruits, such as apples or

blueberries\sgrains, at least half of which
should be whole grains
fat-free or low-fat dairy products
low-fat protein sources, such as chicken,
fish, and soy
healthful oil, such as olive or canola oil
water, tea, or coffee
Cruciferous veggies
Cruciferous vegetables are members of the
Brassica genus. They include:

broccoli\scabbage
cauliflower\sbok choy\skale
Research from 2014Trusted Source shows
that cruciferous veggies may be useful to
persons with leukemia. Researchers
discovered that components in cruciferous
vegetables, such as sulforaphane, might
prevent the spread of some forms of
leukemia.

But scientists discovered that the quantity of
sulforaphane required to effect leukemia
was more than a person would be able to

take through diet alone. Additionally, researchers performed the investigation on samples outside the human body. Further study is essential to discover if sulforaphane is beneficial in treating leukemia in people.

Neutropenic diet
Cancer treatments may impair the immune system and raise the risk of foodborne diseases.

Neutropenia is a disorder that happens when a person has too few neutrophils, a kind of white blood cell for fighting infections. Low neutrophil numbers increase the risk of infections.

Neutropenia is a frequent side effect

Trusted Source of chemotherapy, a sort of cancer treatment. A doctor may prescribe a neutropenic diet for someone who has neutropenia. A neutropenic diet entails eliminating specific items to prevent exposure to microorganisms, such as:

raw or undercooked meat\sraw or undercooked seafood and shellfish, including sushi and sashimi\sunpasteurized liquids, such as fruit juice, milk, or raw milk yogurt\ssoft cheese produced from unpasteurized milk\suncooked or unpasteurized egg, and foods that include it\srefrigerated pâté or deli meats, such as dry-cured uncooked salami\sraw sprouts, such as alfalfa sprouts\sunwashed fruit and vegetables\sfood from buffets or salad bars well water

Some physicians may advocate the neutropenic diet for those who are receiving leukemia therapy. But the LLC argues there is no proof that a neutropenic diet is useful for persons with leukemia. They urge that consumers take care to cook meals safely rather than banning particular food categories.

It is vital to note that various diets will work for different people's requirements. A person should follow their doctor's advice on food and nutrition throughout cancer treatment.

Food, supplements, and vitamins to avoid Certain supplements may interfere with the drugs that treat leukemia, such as:

St John's wort: St John's wort is a supplement that some individuals take for alleviating depression. It may diminish the efficiency of imatinib, which is beneficial for treating chronic myeloid leukemia and Philadelphia-positive acute lymphoblastic leukemia.
Green tea: Some individuals use green tea supplements for weight reduction and relieving digestive issues. Green tea supplements may minimize the effects of bortezomib, a medication for treating acute lymphoblastic leukemia.

Treatments for leukemia may have negative effects, including:

mouth ulcers
diarrhea\shair loss\srash\snausea
vomiting\sfatigue\sloss of
appetite\sneuropathy, which is a kind of
nerve injury
People may wish to avoid foods that might
increase the negative effects of leukemia
therapy, such as trusted Source:

meals rich in fiber or sugar
oily, fatty, or fried meal
extremely hot or very cold meal
milk products
alcohol\sspicy foods
caffeine
apple juice
food sweetened with xylitol or
sorbitol\sfoods that might harm the mouth,
such as those that are crunchy, acidic, or
salty\scitrus fruits
tomatoes with ketchup

Individuals mustn't depend on diet, supplements, or vitamins to treat their leukemia.

FOOD SAFETY

Having a reduced immune system due to leukemia might increase a person's risk of infection. The LLS advises the following guidelines to guarantee food safety:

keeping hands, surfaces, and kitchen objects clean\swashing dishtowels and sponges regularly\srinsing fruits and vegetables before consuming\scutting away any bruised or broken areas of fruits and vegetables\sremoving outer leaves on heads of cabbage and lettuce
utilizing different cutting boards, plates, and tools for preparing raw or cooked meat\savoiding washing raw meat before cooking
thawing frozen foods in a refrigerator or microwave rather than putting them on a

counter\smarinating food in the refrigerator\susing a food thermometer to make sure meat is properly cooked\sensuring food is cooked all the way through before eating

When to consult a doctor

People who have leukemia should always talk with their doctor before modifying their diet. Making unexpected dietary changes may influence health and well-being. If a person has any worries regarding particular meals, they should discuss them with their doctor.

This includes:

persons who are having cancer treatment\spregnant women\syoung children\solder adults

Freshly squeezed fruit and vegetable juices may not have gone through the pasteurization process. As a consequence, individuals could have an increased chance of harboring pathogens. People with less effective or suppressed immune systems could have a more severe response to the impacts of infectious pathogens.

Patients following a low microbial diet on the recommendation of a doctor should avoid unpasteurized fruit and vegetable juices unless they are homemade.

Summary

Cancer is a category of deadly illnesses that are caused by genetic alterations in your cells. Abnormal cancer cells may proliferate fast and create tumors.

Risk factors include smoking, drinking alcohol, a lack of physical exercise, a poor diet, having a high BMI, and contracting certain viruses and bacteria that may contribute to getting cancer.

Screenings may help find cancer early when it is simpler to treat. The treatment strategy and prognosis for persons with cancer might vary on the kind of cancer, the stage at which it is detected, and their age and general health.

Nutritionists advocate a modest and balanced diet for leukemia. A nourishing balancing diet helps in the treatment and quick recovery of cancer patients notably leukemia, it helps with side effects and lowers the chance of problems while receiving treatment.

People receiving treatment for leukemia should avoid some supplements, such as St John's wort. Additionally, many meals might increase the negative effects of leukemia therapy, such as spicy or fatty foods. People should consult with their doctor if they have any concerns about particular meals.

When preparing and storing food, people with leukemia should be careful to follow food safety guidelines. This can reduce their likelihood of developing an illness or infection

BENEFITS

Carrot juice is very nutritious and may be good for avoiding a variety of health issues. We examine these prospective advantages in greater depth below.

Leukemia
More study is required to validate this, but carrot juice may have a future role in leukemia therapy.

In one study, researchers looked at the impact of carrot juice extracts on leukemia cells. The carrot juice extracts induced the leukemia cells to self-destruct and interrupted their cell cycle.

Although it is unlikely to become a solo therapy for leukemia, carrots may be an excellent dietary option for patients with this illness.

Breast cancer

women who survived breast cancer looked
studied the influence of carrot juice on the
levels of carotenoids, indicators of oxidative
stress, and markers of inflammation in the
blood

Stomach cancer

The antioxidants in carrots may help
prevent stomach cancer.
Carrots contain antioxidants, which may
explain their putative function in cancer
prevention.

Pubity: A new medicine being evaluated for
colorectal cancer has left experts surprised
when it reported a 100 percent success rate.

Dostarlimab- injection is used to treat a
particular form of endometrial cancer
(cancer that starts in the lining of the
uterus) in adults that has progressed or has
returned following treatment with other

chemotherapy medication(s) . Dostarlimab-injection is also used to treat a particular form of solid tumor that has progressed to other regions of the body in individuals who were previously treated inadequately with another chemotherapy medicine and do not have any appropriate treatment alternatives. Dostarlimab-injection is in a family of drugs called monoclonal antibodies. It works by preventing the function of a particular protein in cancer cells. This enables the person's immune system to fight against the cancer cells and helps to decrease tumor development